The New Way of Fertility

Revolutionizing Reproductive Health with Modern Science and Holistic Care

DR. ELVIRA S. GRAVES

TABLE OF CONTENTS

Disclaimer

Overview

The Need for a Novel Fertility Strategy

Parenting is still a very personal and frequently difficult process, even in a world where science and technology are developing at an incredible rate. Many prospective parents encounter a maze of challenges in their pursuit of conception, even in the face of major medical advancements and a wealth of resources. There has never been a more urgent need for a new strategy for fertility that combines cutting-edge research with holistic treatment to offer individuals and couples all-encompassing support.

A variety of physical, psychological, and social elements that affect reproductive health are included in the complex field of fertility. From physiological circumstances to environmental impacts, social issues, and individual lifestyle choices, today's challenges are numerous and intricate. The urgent need for a paradigm shift in fertility care that is based on both cutting-edge research and conventional wisdom is intended to be emphasized in this introduction.

The prevalence of infertility, which impacts millions of individuals and couples globally, is one of the biggest obstacles to modern fertility. A global public health concern, infertility affects an estimated 48 million

couples and 186 million individuals worldwide, according to the World Health Organization (WHO). These startling figures highlight the need for creative solutions that cater to the various requirements of infertile individuals.

Many different and frequently complex variables contribute to infertility, including both male and female ones. Ovarian insufficiency, endometriosis, and polycystic ovary syndrome (PCOS) can all seriously impair a woman's ability to conceive. On the other hand, problems like low sperm count, poor sperm motility, and structural abnormalities are often linked to male infertility. Reproductive success is also significantly influenced by variables like age, lifestyle decisions, and underlying medical issues.

The increasing difficulties with conception in recent years have also been a result of societal changes. Due to changing social standards, educational goals, and career aspirations, delayed childbearing has grown more prevalent. These decisions give people and couples the freedom to follow their dreams, but they also pose biological problems because fertility naturally decreases with age. After the age of 35, a woman's ovarian reserve and egg quality start to fall more sharply, which makes conception more challenging. As men age, their sperm quality and fertility gradually deteriorate as well.

It is impossible to overestimate the psychological and emotional toll that infertility takes. The path to parenthood is frequently paved with emotional upheaval, worry, and anxiety. The social stigma attached to

infertility and the urge to become pregnant can strain relationships and have an impact on mental health. Individuals and couples suffer greatly from the emotional rollercoaster of hope and disappointment interspersed with medical procedures and therapies.

The fertility landscape is further complicated by financial restrictions. Many prospective parents may not be able to afford assisted reproductive technologies (ART), such as in vitro fertilization (IVF). Disparities in reproductive healthcare are caused by the high expense of fertility treatments and differing levels of insurance coverage. Comprehensive and reasonably priced care is desperately needed because this financial strain frequently makes the stress and anxiety related to infertility worse.

Despite these obstacles, each person's and couple's journey to fertility is extremely distinctive and distinct. Case studies and personal tales provide light on the many experiences of individuals traveling this path, emphasizing the tenacity and resolve that define the journey to motherhood. For example, consider the tale of Sarah and John. Following years of unsuccessful attempts at natural conception, they resorted to IVF. The birth of their daughter was the ultimate reward for their tenacious journey, which was filled with highs and lows in terms of their emotions. Their experience serves as a reminder of the value of optimism, encouragement, and creative thinking in the field of fertility.

The story of Maria, who battled PCOS and received multiple treatments before ultimately achieving success through a combination of lifestyle modifications and medical interventions is another moving example. Her experience highlights the need for individualized and thorough fertility techniques and demonstrates the possibilities of fusing modern science with holistic care.

These individual stories are not unique occurrences; rather, they are representative of a larger pattern that demands a reconsideration of our conception of fertility. A bright future lies at the nexus of contemporary science and holistic medicine. The fertility landscape has changed due to advancements in reproductive medicine, such as genetic testing, customized treatments, and state-of-the-art technologies. For those who are infertile, these advancements provide fresh hope by facilitating customized strategies that cater to specific requirements and maximize success rates. But being a parent involves more than just medical procedures. Supporting individuals and couples requires holistic care, which takes into account their physical, mental, and spiritual well. Fertility results can be greatly impacted by lifestyle changes like eating a healthy diet, exercising frequently, and practicing stress reduction. Additionally, complementing advantages that improve general reproductive health are provided by alternative therapies including acupuncture, herbal medicine, and mindfulness exercises.

A cooperative strategy is required to integrate contemporary science with holistic care. To develop complete reproductive methods that meet the specific needs of each person and couple, healthcare professionals, researchers, and holistic practitioners must collaborate. We can transform reproductive health and give people pursuing children a new direction by fusing the benefits of holistic practices with modern developments.

In conclusion, the existing issues and data that characterize the reproductive landscape make it clear that a new approach to fertility is required. Case studies and personal tales demonstrate the tenacity and resolve of people and couples overcoming the challenges of infertility. Adopting a comprehensive and scientifically grounded approach to fertility will empower prospective parents and open the door to a more promising future in reproductive healthcare as we proceed. The goal of this book is to support readers as they set out on the life-changing journey to motherhood by providing them with advice, techniques, and hope.

Section One

Chapter 1: Understanding Fertility

The ability to conceive and maintain a pregnancy is the result of a complex interaction between biological, environmental, and behavioral variables. A detailed understanding of human reproductive anatomy and physiology, men's and women's hormone cycles, and typical fertility problems and causes is necessary to comprehend fertility. Effective fertility methods and therapies are based on this thorough understanding.

The Study of Reproduction
An overview of the anatomy and physiology of the human reproductive system. To promote fertilization and the subsequent development of an embryo, the human reproductive system is precisely constructed to generate, sustain, and transport gametes, which are sperm in males and eggs (ova) in females. Every component of this system is essential to reproduction, underscoring the need to preserve reproductive health.

The reproductive system of women

There are internal and external components that make up the female reproductive system. The mons pubis, labia majora, labia minora, clitoris, and vaginal vestibule are the exterior structures that make up the vulva. These structures contribute to sexual excitement and pleasure while also protecting the interior genital organs.

The uterus, vagina, fallopian tubes, and ovaries are the main reproductive organs found inside the body. On either side of the uterus are tiny, almond-shaped structures called ovaries. They produce eggs and secrete hormones like progesterone and estrogen, which are their two primary roles. An egg develops inside an ovarian follicle during each menstrual cycle and is released during ovulation.

The egg is transported from the ovary to the uterus by the fallopian tubes, sometimes referred to as oviducts. The fallopian tube, where the sperm meets and enters the egg, is where fertilization often takes place.

The pear-shaped organ known as the uterus is where fetal development and embryo implantation take place. The endometrium (inner lining), myometrium (muscular middle layer), and perimetrium (outer layer) make up its three layers. Hormonal changes during the menstrual cycle cause the endometrium to thicken and shed.

The uterus and the outside world are connected by the vagina, a muscular tube. In addition to absorbing sperm during sexual activity, it also facilitates birthing and acts as a conduit for menstrual flow.

The Reproductive System of Men

Sperm production, maintenance, and delivery are the functions of the male reproductive system. It has internal as well as external structures. The scrotum and penis are the exterior structures. The organ used for sperm delivery and sexual activity is the penis. The urethra passes through the middle of it, which is made up of the shaft and the glans.

The testes are located in the scrotum, a pouch that hangs beneath the penis. The main male reproductive organs, the testes, are in charge of generating testosterone and sperm. The seminiferous tubules in the testes are where sperm generation takes place. Sperm mature after production and are kept in the epididymis, a coiled tube located behind each testis.

Sperm passes through the vas deferens to the ejaculatory ducts during ejaculation, where they combine with seminal fluid from the prostate gland and seminal vesicles. During ejaculation, this mixture becomes semen, which is released through the urethra.

Women's and Men's Hormonal Cycles

In both men and women, hormones are essential for controlling the reproductive processes. These hormones control the maturation, release, and development of gametes as well as the process by which the reproductive organs are ready for implantation and fertilization.

Women's Hormonal Cycle

The monthly hormonal cycle known as the menstrual cycle primes the female body for pregnancy. It is separated into multiple stages, each of which is distinguished by particular physiological occurrences and hormonal alterations.

1. Menstrual Phase: This phase, which lasts for three to seven days, signifies the start of the cycle. Menstrual bleeding is the result of the uterine lining being shed.

2. Follicular Phase: This stage lasts until ovulation and crosses over into the menstrual phase. Gonadotropin-releasing hormone (GnRH), which is released by the brain during this phase, causes the pituitary gland to release follicle-stimulating hormone (FSH). Ovarian follicle development and maturation are aided by FSH. The endometrium thickens due to the production of estrogen by developing follicles.

3. Ovulation: A spike in luteinizing hormone (LH) from the pituitary gland causes ovulation, which happens about the middle of the cycle. The developed follicle releases its egg into the fallopian tube as a result of this LH surge.

4. Luteal Phase: The corpus luteum, which secretes progesterone, develops from the burst follicle following ovulation. In order to prepare the endometrial lining for the possible implantation of a fertilized egg, progesterone keeps it healthy. The corpus luteum degenerates in the absence of fertilization, which lowers progesterone levels and causes menstruation.

Men's Hormonal Cycle

The male reproductive system functions continuously, in contrast to the female reproductive system's cyclical nature. But hormonal interactions, mainly involving the hypothalamus, pituitary gland, and testes, also control it.

1. Hypothalamic-Pituitary-Gonadal Axis: The pituitary gland secretes FSH and LH in response to the hypothalamus' production of GnRH. While LH increases the production of testosterone by the Leydig cells, FSH acts on the Sertoli cells in the testes to enhance spermatogenesis.

2. Production of Testosterone: The main male sex hormone, testosterone is in charge of the development of secondary sexual traits in men, including body hair, a deeper voice, and more muscle mass. Additionally, it is essential for spermatogenesis and libido maintenance.

Typical Fertility Problems and Their Causes

Numerous variables that impact one or both partners can result in fertility problems. Diagnosing and treating reproductive problems requires an understanding of these prevalent problems and their causes.

Problems with Female Fertility

Disorders of Ovulation

A primary cause of infertility in women is ovulatory disorders, which arise from abnormalities in the regular ovulation process. Hypothalamic amenorrhea and polycystic ovarian syndrome (PCOS) are two of the most prevalent ovulatory illnesses.

PCOS, or polycystic ovary syndrome, is a hormonal condition marked by polycystic ovaries, irregular menstruation periods, and elevated testosterone levels. Conception might be challenging for women with PCOS because they may not ovulate consistently and have irregular or delayed menstrual cycles. Although the precise origin of PCOS is unknown, a mix of environmental and genetic factors is thought to be involved. Women with PCOS frequently have insulin resistance, which raises insulin levels and can further interfere with ovulation by increasing testosterone production. Weight gain, acne, hirsutism (excessive hair growth), and thinning hair on the scalp are typical symptoms. PCOS-related infertility can be treated with drugs such as clomiphene citrate to induce ovulation, dietary and activity modifications to increase insulin sensitivity, and, if required, assisted reproductive technologies (ART).

Hypothalamic Amenorrhea: This condition happens when the brain region known as the hypothalamus, which controls reproductive hormones, ceases to release gonadotropin-releasing hormone (GnRH). Follicle-stimulating hormone (FSH) and luteinizing hormone (LH), which are essential for ovulation, are not secreted by the pituitary gland as a result of this disturbance. Excessive physical stress, dramatic weight loss, low body fat, or psychological stress can all cause hypothalamic amenorrhea. Those with eating disorders, athletes, and dancers are more vulnerable. Amenorrhea, or the lack of menstruation, and low estrogen levels are among the symptoms. To restore normal hypothalamic function and ovulation, treatment entails addressing the underlying reason, which may include decreasing physical activity, gaining weight, or managing stress.

Endometriosis

The disorder known as endometriosis occurs when the endometrium, the tissue that normally lines the lining of the uterus, develops outside of it. The ovaries, fallopian tubes, uterine exteriors, and other pelvic organs might all have ectopic endometrial tissue. Pain, inflammation, and the development of adhesions, or scar tissue, are all possible side effects of endometriosis. Although the precise etiology of endometriosis is unknown, possibilities include immune system problems, hereditary factors, and retrograde menstruation, which is the movement of menstrual blood backward via the fallopian tubes into the pelvic cavity. Chronic pelvic pain, painful menstruation (dysmenorrhea), pain during sexual activity, and infertility are all signs of endometriosis. Additionally, gastrointestinal symptoms including bloating and constipation, as well as heavy menstrual bleeding, may result from the illness. Deformed pelvic architecture, inflammation, and compromised ovulation and fallopian tube function can all affect fertility.
A pelvic exam, imaging tests such as MRI or ultrasound, and laparoscopy—a surgical procedure in which a camera is placed into the pelvis to view and biopsy the ectopic tissue—are frequently used to diagnose endometriosis. Nonsteroidal anti-inflammatory medication (NSAID) pain management, hormonal therapy to lessen or stop menstruation, and surgical excision of endometrial implants and

adhesions are among the available treatment options. ART, such as IVF, may be advised for women whose infertility is caused by endometriosis.

Tubal Elements

When the fallopian tubes are obstructed or injured, the sperm and egg cannot meet, resulting in tubal factor infertility. In order to catch the ovulated egg, facilitate fertilization, and move the fertilized egg to the uterus for implantation, the fallopian tubes are essential. Several illnesses, such as infections, pelvic inflammatory disease (PID), and prior procedures, can cause tubal damage. Sexually transmitted infections (STIs) such as gonorrhea and chlamydia are frequently the cause of Pelvic Inflammatory Disease (PID), an illness of the female reproductive system. The infection may cause the fallopian tubes to become inflamed and scarred, which may obstruct or harm them. Pelvic pain, fever, irregular vaginal discharge, and discomfort while urination or sexual activity are all signs of PID. To avoid long-term issues such as tubal infertility, early diagnosis, and antibiotic treatment are essential. Prior Surgeries: Scar tissue formation and adhesions may result from pelvic organ-related surgeries, such as appendectomy, ovarian cyst removal, or ectopic pregnancy surgery. The fallopian tubes may become deformed or obstructed as a result of these adhesions.

illnesses: Infertility can also result from non-sexually transmitted illnesses that impact the fallopian tubes, such as TB. These infections can occasionally be asymptomatic, which makes early detection difficult.

A hysterosalpingography (HSG) test, which employs X-ray imaging to examine the fallopian tubes and uterus after injecting a contrast dye, is commonly used to diagnose tubal factor infertility. Depending on the extent of the tubal injury, treatment options may involve either surgical tube repair or ART, such as IVF, which involves external fertilization.

Abnormalities of the Uterus

The capacity to maintain a pregnancy and facilitate implantation can be hampered by structural abnormalities in the uterus. These anomalies may be acquired (occurring later in life) or congenital (existing from birth). Benign tumors called fibroids develop inside the uterine wall. Depending on where they are, their size and location may have an impact on fertility. The most likely to disrupt implantation and pregnancy are submucosal fibroids, which proliferate into the uterus. Heavy menstrual flow, pelvic pain, and pressure on the bladder or colon are signs of fibroids. Medication to control symptoms, non-invasive techniques such as uterine artery embolization, and surgical excision by myomectomy are available treatment options.

Polyps: Polyps are growths that appear on the endometrium, the uterine lining. Their size might vary, and they can lead to infertility, spotting in between periods, and unpredictable menstrual bleeding. Hysteroscopy or ultrasound can be used to diagnose polyps, and surgery can be used to remove them.

Congenital Malformations: Pregnancy outcomes and fertility may be impacted by congenital uterine abnormalities such as a bicornuate uterus, which is a heart-shaped uterus with two cavities, or a septate uterus, which is a uterine cavity separated by a septum. Imaging procedures like MRIs, hysteroscopies, and ultrasounds are frequently used to diagnose these abnormalities. To increase fertility and lower the chance of pregnancy difficulties, surgery may be advised.

Reduced Ovarian Supply

Fertility may be impacted by diminished ovarian reserve (DOR), which is defined as a reduction in the number and quality of a woman's eggs. Age, medical treatments like chemotherapy or radiation therapy, or procedures that remove all or part of the ovaries can all contribute to DOR.

Age-Related Decline: As women become older, their ovaries naturally produce fewer eggs and the quality of those that are left deteriorates. After the age of 35, this drop gets more pronounced, making it harder to conceive and raising the chance of miscarriage and fetal chromosome abnormalities.

Medical Treatments: Ovarian damage and ovarian reserve can result from treatments for specific medical disorders, such as cancer. Radiation and chemotherapy can be especially detrimental to ovarian function. Before beginning therapy, women undergoing these procedures can think about fertility preservation options including freezing eggs or embryos.

Diagnosis and Treatment: Antral follicle count (AFC), as determined by ultrasound, and blood tests measuring anti-Müllerian hormone (AMH) and follicle-stimulating hormone (FSH) levels are frequently used to diagnose DOR. IVF, fertility drugs to stimulate the ovaries, and, if required, donor egg use are treatment options for women with DOR.

Problems with Male Fertility

Disorders of Sperm Production

The amount, quality, and functionality of sperm are all impacted by sperm production abnormalities, which can have a major effect on male fertility. Asthenozoospermia, teratozoospermia, and oligospermia are common abnormalities of sperm production.

A lower-than-normal concentration of sperm in the ejaculate is known as low sperm count (oligospermia). Hormonal imbalances, genetic disorders, infections, and lifestyle decisions are just a few of the causes. Low sperm count is diagnosed through a semen examination, and treatment options may include lifestyle changes, hormonally addressing drugs, and assisted reproductive methods such as IVF or IUI.

Poor Sperm Motility (Asthenozoospermia): This condition is characterized by decreased sperm motility, which makes it difficult for the sperm to swim and get to the egg. Genetics, diseases, lifestyle choices, and sperm structural anomalies can all contribute to this syndrome. Changes in lifestyle, medicine, and ART like as intracytoplasmic sperm injection (ICSI), which involves injecting a single sperm into an egg, are possible treatment options.

Teratozoospermia, or aberrant sperm morphology, is typified by a significant proportion of sperm with atypical shapes. The size and form of sperm might affect their capacity to fertilize an egg; this is known as sperm morphology. Teratozoospermia can be caused by genetic defects, infections, environmental pollutants, and lifestyle choices like smoking and binge drinking. It may be more difficult for sperm to swim effectively and enter the egg if they have an irregular form. Treatment options include changing one's lifestyle, taking care of underlying health issues, and using assisted reproductive technologies like ICSI, which involves injecting an egg with a single, healthy-looking sperm.

Varicocele

Similar to varicose veins in the legs, a varicocele is an enlargement of the veins in the scrotum. About 15% of men and up to 40% of men with infertility suffer from this illness, which is one of the most prevalent reasons for male infertility. Because varicoceles raise the temperature in the scrotum, they can reduce the quantity and quality of sperm produced by the testicles. Vein enlargement that is palpable or visible, a testicular lump, swelling, or a dull, agonizing pain that gets worse with movement or extended standing are all signs of varicocele. Surgical techniques such as varicocelectomy, which involves cutting off the afflicted veins to reroute blood flow and enhance sperm production, are available as treatment alternatives.

Disorders of Ejaculation

Fertility may be impacted by ejaculatory abnormalities, which can hinder sperm from being appropriately ejected from the body. When semen enters the bladder during ejaculation rather than exiting from the penis, this is known as retrograde ejaculation. As a result, during an orgasm, little to no semen may be discharged. Retrograde ejaculation can be brought on by nerve damage from diseases like diabetes or multiple sclerosis, bladder or prostate procedures, and some drugs. Options for treatment could include taking drugs to make the muscles in the neck of the bladder stronger, treating underlying illnesses, or using assisted reproductive methods to get sperm straight from the testes or bladder.

Other conditions affecting ejaculation include:

Ejaculation that happens earlier than intended, frequently before or soon after penetration, is known as premature ejaculation. This condition can affect a person's ability to procreate. Medication, counseling, and behavioral strategies may all be used in treatment.
The inability to ejaculate, or anejaculation, can be brought on by psychological issues, spinal cord injury, or damage to the nerves. Medication, addressing the underlying reason, or assisted reproductive methods including sperm harvesting straight from the testicles are among possible forms of treatment.

Factors related to genetics
By altering sperm production and function, genetic defects can have a major effect on male fertility.
A guy born with an extra X chromosome (47, XXY instead of the normal 46, XY) is said to have Klinefelter syndrome, a genetic disorder. Smaller testicles, decreased testosterone levels, and decreased sperm production are all possible outcomes of this disorder. Learning disabilities decreased muscular mass, and gynecomastia (enlarged breast tissue) are some of the symptoms that men with Klinefelter syndrome may encounter. Assisted reproductive methods like testicular sperm extraction (TESE) in conjunction with ICSI can occasionally aid achieve pregnancy, even though men with Klinefelter syndrome may have decreased fertility.

Y Chromosome Microdeletions: These are genetic material deletions on the Y chromosome that can impact genes that are essential for the creation of sperm. Male infertility is frequently caused by Y

chromosomal microdeletions, which can result in oligospermia or azoospermia (the total lack of sperm in the ejaculate). These deletions can be detected by genetic testing, and ICSI in conjunction with sperm retrieval methods may be a therapy option.

Lifestyle and Environmental Factors

Male fertility and sperm quality can be greatly impacted by environmental and lifestyle variables. Typical elements consist of:

Exposure to Toxins: Pesticides, heavy metals, and industrial chemicals are examples of environmental toxins that can harm sperm DNA and lower sperm quality. These effects can be lessened by limiting exposure to these poisons, using protective gear, and leading a healthy lifestyle.

Smoking: Sperm motility, morphology, and count are all linked to tobacco use. Cigarette toxins have the potential to damage sperm DNA and induce oxidative stress. Overall fertility and sperm quality can be enhanced by quitting smoking.

Excessive Alcohol Use: Drinking too much alcohol can cause testicular shrinkage, lower testosterone levels, and interfere with sperm formation. Sperm quality can be improved by reducing alcohol use or refraining from it completely.

Obesity: Hormonal imbalances associated with obesity, such as elevated estrogen and decreased testosterone, can have a detrimental effect on sperm production. Fertility and hormonal balance can be enhanced by losing weight with a healthy diet and consistent exercise.

Heat Exposure: Extended exposure to high temperatures can raise scrotal temperature and reduce sperm production. Examples of this include frequent usage of hot baths, saunas, or tight-fitting

undergarments. Wearing loose-fitting clothing and minimizing heat exposure can assist in maintaining the ideal testicular temperature. *Drug Use:* Recreational drug use, including cocaine, marijuana, and anabolic steroids, can hurt the quality and quantity of sperm. Fertility results can be improved by abstaining from or stopping the usage of these drugs.

Unaccounted for and Combined Infertility

Combination infertility is a condition in which both couples may have contributing causes to infertility. Furthermore, unexplained infertility happens when a comprehensive evaluation yields no identifiable cause. This category emphasizes the intricacy of fertility and the requirement for thorough evaluation and individualized care. Addressing fertility concerns starts with a thorough understanding of the science of reproduction, men's and women's hormone cycles, and typical reproductive problems and causes. With this information, individuals and couples are more equipped to seek out the right therapies, whether they be holistic approaches, lifestyle changes, or medical treatments. We are getting closer to transforming reproductive health and giving individuals pursuing children fresh hope as we investigate and combine contemporary science with holistic care.

Chapter 2: A Comprehensive Perspective on Fertility

The process of becoming fertile involves a complex fusion of the mind, body, and spirit rather than just a biological one. The holistic perspective provides a supplemental strategy that takes into account the full person, even if contemporary science has made great progress in comprehending and treating fertility problems. A thorough foundation for maximizing reproductive health is provided by integrating the mind, body, and spirit; acknowledging the influence of lifestyle, nutrition, and stress; and respecting both conventional and alternative medical viewpoints.

Combining Spirit, Body, and Mind
The interdependence of emotional, physical, and spiritual health is emphasized by the holistic approach to fertility. This viewpoint is based on the knowledge that our mental, emotional, and spiritual practices have a significant impact on our physical well-being, including our ability to conceive.

Reproductive health is greatly impacted by the mind-body connection, which is an inseparable bond between the two. Menstrual cycles, sperm production, and hormonal balance can all be impacted by stress, worry, and negative emotions. On the other hand, mindfulness exercises, relaxation techniques and pleasant emotions can improve fertility and hormonal balance. It has been demonstrated that methods including yoga, mindfulness meditation, and cognitive-behavioral therapy (CBT) can lower stress and enhance fertility. These techniques support people in managing stress, developing a positive outlook, and improving their general well-being.

Spiritual Well-Being: During the fertility process, spirituality—which is characterized as a feeling of belonging to something bigger than oneself—can offer emotional support and fortitude. This could entail religious activities for some people, but it could also refer to a more general sense of purpose and a bond with the natural world or community for others. Praying, meditating, or spending time in nature are examples of spiritual activities that help lower stress, promote emotional health, and cultivate a sense of calm. Additionally, spirituality can help people traverse the difficulties and uncertainties of the reproductive journey with more ease by providing a sense of hope and trust. Understanding each person's or couple's particular needs and experiences is essential to integrating mind, body, and spirit. A more humane and successful route to fertility may be offered by customized strategies that respect these interrelated factors.

The Effects of Stress, Nutrition, and Lifestyle on Fertility
Stress levels, food preferences, and lifestyle decisions all have a significant impact on reproductive health. Fertility and general well-being can be improved by implementing stress-reduction techniques, a balanced diet, and a healthy lifestyle.

Lifestyle Decisions: The cornerstone of maximizing fertility is adopting a healthy lifestyle. It is crucial to engage in regular physical activity, get enough sleep, and abstain from dangerous substances like tobacco, excessive alcohol, and recreational drugs. Exercise promotes hormonal equilibrium, lowers stress, and increases circulation. Striking a balance is crucial, though, because too much exercise might impair fertility by upsetting menstrual cycles and hormonal balance.

Nutrition and Diet: Maintaining reproductive health requires a diet high in nutrients. Both men and women need essential nutrients such as antioxidants, omega-3 fatty acids, iron, zinc, and folate. Folate is necessary for DNA synthesis and cellular activity and can be found in leafy greens, legumes, and fortified meals. Lean meats, legumes, and fortified cereals are good sources of iron, which promotes healthy blood flow and oxygen delivery. Nuts, seeds, and whole grains include zinc, which is essential for immunological and hormone production. Flaxseeds, walnuts, and fatty fish are good sources of omega-3 fatty acids, which help maintain hormonal balance and lower inflammation. Antioxidants, which are found in fruits, vegetables, nuts, and seeds, support reproductive health by shielding cells from oxidative stress.

A balanced diet for women promotes healthy eggs, hormone production, and regular menstrual periods. Men's sperm generation, motility, and morphology are all improved by an adequate diet. Improved reproductive outcomes have been linked to particular food patterns, such as the Mediterranean diet. This diet offers a wide range of nutrients to support reproductive health, with an emphasis on whole grains, fruits, vegetables, lean proteins, and healthy fats.

Stress management: By upsetting the hormonal balance and influencing the reproductive organs, long-term stress can have a major negative influence on fertility. Cortisol and other stress hormones are released as part of the body's stress reaction, and this can disrupt the synthesis of reproductive hormones like testosterone, progesterone, and estrogen. Stress can further affect fertility by altering decisions and behaviors linked to sleep, exercise, and nutrition.

Optimizing fertility requires the use of effective stress management strategies. By encouraging relaxation and strengthening emotional resilience, mindfulness exercises like yoga and meditation can lower stress. Exercise is another powerful stress-reduction strategy since it lowers cortisol levels and releases endorphins. Hobbies, time spent with loved ones, and getting help from support groups or counselors can also help manage stress and enhance general well-being.

Perspectives on Conventional and Alternative Medicine

Modern reproductive therapies can benefit from the useful insights and practices provided by traditional and alternative medical viewpoints. These methods target the underlying causes of infertility problems and acknowledge the need for holistic care.

For decades, the ancient medical system known as Traditional Chinese Medicine (TCM) has been utilized to promote fertility. It includes several techniques, such as food treatment, herbal medicine, and acupuncture. TCM stresses the body's energy (qi) balance and sees fertility as a sign of general health. Thin needles are inserted into particular body locations during acupuncture, a crucial part of TCM, to encourage the flow of qi and aid in healing. According to research, acupuncture can increase fertility by regulating hormone balance, lowering stress levels, and improving blood flow to the reproductive organs.

Another essential component of TCM is herbal medicine, which uses plant-based treatments to promote reproductive health. Red clover, chaste tree, and dong quai are common plants that are thought to boost fertility, control menstrual cycles, and improve the quality of eggs. In TCM, dietary therapy is centered on providing the body with nutrient-dense meals that balance the body's vitality and promote reproductive health.

Ayurveda: For optimum health, the Indian traditional medical system of Ayurveda stresses the harmony of the mind, body, and spirit. Herbal treatment, dietary advice, and lifestyle changes are all part of Ayurvedic fertility methods. Ashwagandha, Shatavari, and guggul are among the herbs that are frequently used to promote reproductive health because they balance hormones, lower stress levels, and increase general vitality. A balanced diet full of whole foods, healthy fats, and spices like ginger and turmeric, which have anti-inflammatory and antioxidant qualities, is also emphasized by Ayurveda. To preserve equilibrium and encourage fertility, lifestyle choices like consistent exercise, yoga, and meditation are essential.

The alternative medical practice of homeopathy is founded on the idea that "like cures like." In order to promote the body's natural healing processes, very diluted chemicals are used. Fertility homeopathic treatments are customized based on each person's particular symptoms and constitution. Sepia, pulsatilla, and sulfur are common treatments that are thought to alleviate mental stress, hormone imbalances, and other fertility-affecting variables.

Naturopathy: Naturopathy stresses the body's innate capacity for self-healing and is a comprehensive approach to healthcare. To promote reproductive health, naturopathic practitioners combine herbal medicine, nutritional and lifestyle changes, and other natural therapies. Identifying and treating the underlying causes of health problems, encouraging healthy lifestyle choices, and utilizing natural remedies to aid in the body's healing processes are all fundamental tenets of naturopathy. Naturopathic therapies for fertility may involve lifestyle changes to lower stress and improve general well-being, herbal medicines to maintain hormonal balance, and dietary advice to guarantee sufficient intake of vital nutrients. To support reproductive health, naturopathy also highlights the significance of environmental factors, such as lowering exposure to pollutants.

The study of the relationships between mental, emotional, and physical health is known as mind-body medicine. Stress reduction, mental well-being and physical health are all aided by methods like mindfulness meditation, relaxation exercises, and biofeedback. In terms of fertility, mind-body medicine can assist people in lowering stress, enhancing hormonal balance, and managing the emotional difficulties of the reproductive process. Techniques like progressive muscle relaxation, which eases physical tension, and guided imagery, which entails imagining favorable outcomes, can be very helpful.

A complete approach to reproductive health can be achieved by combining contemporary fertility therapies with traditional and alternative medical viewpoints. Individuals and couples can maximize their fertility and general well-being by taking care of their minds, body, and spirit as well as understanding the effects of stress, food, and lifestyle choices. This all-encompassing perspective offers a kind and practical route to parenting, enabling people to take control of their reproductive health and go through the conception process more confidently and easily. We get closer to a more comprehensive and individualized approach to fertility therapy as we investigate and incorporate these many viewpoints. This chapter lays the groundwork for comprehending the interdependence of the mind, body, and spirit; the importance of lifestyle, nutrition, and stress; and the insightful information provided by both conventional and alternative medical viewpoints. We can transform reproductive health and give individuals pursuing family fresh hope by adopting this comprehensive viewpoint.

Section Two

Chapter 3: Fertility and Modern Science

Reproductive medicine has reached previously unheard-of heights thanks to modern science, which has given individuals and couples facing infertility issues creative answers and hope. This chapter explores the amazing developments in reproductive medicine, with a particular emphasis on new technology and fertility therapies that have completely changed how we see and treat infertility.

Developments in the Field of Reproductive Medicine
The past few decades have seen a considerable evolution in reproductive medicine due to advances in genetics, human biology, and the creation of innovative medical technology. These developments have increased

the options accessible to individuals and couples looking to conceive, in addition to improving our capacity to identify and treat infertility.

The creation of assisted reproductive technologies (ART) is among the most important developments in reproductive medicine. A range of medical treatments intended to treat infertility and aid in conception are together referred to as ART. In vitro fertilization (IVF), the most well-known ART technique, entails fertilizing an egg with sperm outside of the body and then implanting the resulting embryo into the uterus. IVF has experienced several advancements and improvements since its debut, increasing its accessibility and success rates.

Hormonal therapy is another important development in reproductive medicine. Infertility is frequently caused by hormonal imbalances, and hormonal treatments have shown great promise in controlling ovulation and enhancing reproductive results. Medications including gonadotropins, letrozole, and clomiphene citrate are frequently used to induce ovulation in women who have irregular menstrual periods or anovulation. By encouraging the development and maturity of ovarian follicles, these drugs raise the chances of a successful pregnancy.

Reproductive medicine has advanced significantly as a result of surgical procedures in addition to hormonal therapy. Laparoscopy and hysteroscopy are two examples of minimally invasive surgical procedures used to identify and treat a variety of diseases that may impair fertility. To visualize and treat diseases like endometriosis, pelvic adhesions, and ovarian cysts, laparoscopy entails creating tiny incisions in the belly to introduce a camera and surgical tools. A camera is inserted through the cervix into the uterus during a hysteroscopy to identify and treat uterine abnormalities like adhesions, fibroids, and polyps.

Fertility preservation has been transformed by cryopreservation, which involves freezing and storing reproductive cells and tissues. With the use of this technology, people can save their fertility for later use, which is especially advantageous for patients receiving treatments like radiation or chemotherapy that could harm their reproductive system. Eggs, sperm, and embryos can be stored by cryopreservation, giving individuals and couples the option to become pregnant later.

Another new area of reproductive medicine that has attracted a lot of interest is reproductive immunology. Investigating how immunological variables may lead to infertility and recurrent pregnancy loss, this field looks at the involvement of the immune system in fertility and pregnancy. Intravenous immunoglobulin (IVIG) therapy and corticosteroids are two treatments that target immune responses and have demonstrated promise in improving reproductive outcomes for people with immunological disorders.

Innovations in Fertility Technologies and Treatments
Numerous revolutionary developments in reproductive technologies and therapies over the last few decades have changed how we see infertility and increased the likelihood of a successful pregnancy.

The process of removing immature eggs from the ovaries and developing them in a lab prior to fertilization is known as in vitro maturation, or IVM. By minimizing the requirement for hormonal stimulation, this method lowers the risk of ovarian hyperstimulation syndrome (OHSS) and increases the accessibility and safety of fertility treatments for women with particular disorders. Women who have polycystic ovarian syndrome (PCOS) or are at risk of developing OHSS benefit most from IVM.

Before implantation, embryos are screened for genetic abnormalities using a procedure called preimplantation genetic testing, or PGT. This testing lowers the risk of genetic abnormalities and increases the likelihood of successful pregnancies. Preimplantation genetic screening (PGS) for chromosomal abnormalities and preimplantation genetic diagnosis (PGD) for single-gene disorders are both included in PGT. PGT increases IVF success rates and helps stop the spread of genetic illnesses by choosing genetically healthy embryos.

Ovarian Tissue Transplantation: This procedure entails taking ovarian tissue, freezing it, and then re-implantation. When women are receiving treatments like chemotherapy or radiation that could harm their ovaries, this method is utilized to preserve their fertility. For women who want to maintain their ability to procreate, ovarian tissue transplantation is a feasible alternative because it can restore fertility and hormonal function. Young cancer patients who want to continue being fertile after treatment have found this therapy to be especially helpful.

Three-Parent IVF: Also referred to as mitochondrial replacement therapy (MRT), three-parent IVF entails substituting healthy mitochondrial DNA from a donor for damaged mitochondrial DNA in an egg. This method is employed to stop the spread of mitochondrial illnesses, which are hereditary conditions brought on by mutations in the DNA of the mitochondria. Three-parent IVF guarantees that the child is free of certain genetic disorders by utilizing mitochondrial DNA from a healthy donor. Families with mitochondrial abnormalities now have more options thanks to this innovative approach.

Reproductive medicine is changing as a result of artificial intelligence (AI) and machine learning, which improve decision-making and facilitate the study of big data. These technologies can determine which embryos are the most viable, estimate the success rates of ART, and customize treatment regimens. Clinicians are using AI-driven tools to optimize reproductive treatments and increase success rates, such as predictive models for treatment outcomes and algorithms for rating embryos. The use of AI in reproductive medicine has enormous potential for improving fertility treatment in the future.

Stem Cell Therapy: This new discipline has the potential to completely transform fertility treatments. The use of stem cells to repair ovarian tissue, enhance the quality of eggs, and increase fertility in women with reduced ovarian reserve or premature ovarian failure is still being investigated. Additionally, by enhancing sperm production and rebuilding testicular tissue, stem cell therapy may be able to solve male infertility. Even though it is still in the experimental phase, stem cell therapy presents intriguing prospects for reproductive health in the future.

Time-Lapse Imaging: This technique is used in IVF to continuously track the development of the embryo. Using this method, embryologists can watch the embryos grow and develop without disturbing them by taking pictures of them at regular intervals. Using time-lapse imaging, embryologists can choose the most viable embryos for transfer by learning important details about the developmental patterns of the embryos. By improving embryo selection, this method has been demonstrated to increase IVF success rates.

Egg and Sperm Donation: For people and couples who are unable to conceive using their own gametes, egg and sperm donation offers viable possibilities. IVF can use donor sperm and eggs to get pregnant. The use of donor gametes has given infertile people fresh hope and increased their options for starting a family. The best quality and compatibility for successful outcomes are guaranteed by advancements in donor screening and matching. Furthermore, the availability of donor gametes has made different families—such as same-sex couples and single parents—more accessible and inclusive.

For people or couples who are unable to conceive or carry a pregnancy to term, surrogacy is utilizing a gestational carrier to bring a pregnancy to term. Traditional surrogacy, which uses the surrogate's egg, and gestational surrogacy, which uses the intended parents' or donor's egg, are two new choices for starting a family thanks to advancements in surrogacy. Surrogacy agreements must take ethics and legal issues into account to protect the rights and welfare of all parties. For same-sex male couples and those with medical issues like uterine factor infertility, surrogacy has emerged as a feasible alternative.

Fertility Preservation: For those who choose to postpone motherhood or who are receiving medical treatments that may impact their fertility, fertility preservation methods including freezing eggs, sperm, and embryos offer alternatives. For those undergoing cancer treatments, autoimmune illnesses, or other conditions that affect reproductive health, these methods provide flexibility and hope. The success rates of fertility preservation and subsequent ART operations have increased due to advancements in cryopreservation technology. By offering choices for family planning and job considerations, fertility preservation has also given people the ability to take charge of their reproductive futures.

Genetic Testing and Counseling: These days, genetic testing and counseling are essential parts of reproductive treatment. Assessing a person's or a couple's genetic risk factors and offering knowledge, support, and direction on reproductive options are all part of genetic counseling. To maximize reproductive results, genetic testing can be done on both potential parents and embryos. The discovery of genetic mutations, chromosomal abnormalities, and other genetic factors that may affect fertility is made possible by techniques like whole-genome sequencing and next-generation sequencing (NGS), which offer comprehensive insights into an individual's genetic composition. Individuals and couples are empowered to make knowledgeable decisions regarding their family planning and reproductive health through genetic counseling and testing.

The landscape of fertility care has changed as a result of advancements in reproductive medicine, fertility treatments, and technologies, which have given infertile individuals and couples new hope and opportunities. By combining individualized care with medical therapies, these advancements provide a complete strategy for treating infertility and maximizing reproductive outcomes. We are getting closer to transforming reproductive health and giving people pursuing family fresh hope as we investigate and incorporate these developments. The contribution of contemporary science to fertility is evidence of the strength of creativity and the possibility of new findings that will continue to influence reproductive medicine.

The Function of Genetic Testing in Fertility
Because it offers priceless insights into the genetic factors that can affect fertility, genetic testing has emerged as a crucial tool in the field of reproductive medicine. Prospective parents and medical professionals can detect genetic abnormalities, evaluate risks, and make well-informed decisions to improve reproductive outcomes by using several types of genetic testing. Carrier screening is the process of checking people for particular genetic variants that they might have but not show. People from communities where specific genetic problems are highly prevalent or those with a family history of genetic illnesses should pay particular attention to this kind of screening. For instance, carrier screening can identify diseases such as Tay-Sachs disease, sickle cell anemia, and

cystic fibrosis. Couples can investigate techniques like preimplantation genetic testing (PGT) to choose embryos free of these mutations and learn about the chances of spreading genetic illnesses to their children by knowing their carrier status.

Preimplantation Genetic Testing (PGT): During an IVF cycle, PGT includes several methods for checking embryos for genetic defects before implantation. By ensuring that only healthy embryos are placed in the uterus, this testing lowers the danger of genetic diseases and increases the likelihood of a successful pregnancy. PGT falls into two primary categories:

Preimplantation genetic diagnosis, or PGD, is a screening method for certain genetic abnormalities brought on by mutations in a single gene. Using PGD, couples who are known to carry certain mutations can choose embryos that are free of the condition.

Preimplantation Genetic Screening (PGS): Also referred to as aneuploidy screening, PGS checks embryos for chromosomal abnormalities that may result in Down syndrome or miscarriage. The probability of a successful pregnancy is increased by PGS, which selects embryos with normal chromosomes.

Molecular Genetics and Next-Generation Sequencing (NGS): By offering thorough insights into a person's genetic composition, developments in molecular genetics and NGS have completely changed genetic testing. These technologies make it possible to detect even the tiniest chromosomal defects and genetic alterations. The complete genome or certain regions of interest can be analyzed using NGS, yielding comprehensive data that can direct individualized reproductive therapies. This degree of accuracy aids in locating genetic variables that could impact fertility and developing customized treatments to deal with them.

Genetic Counseling: In order to help individuals and couples deal with the intricacies of genetic testing, genetic counseling is essential. Genetic counselors use the findings of genetic testing to provide advice, support, and information. In order to maximize fertility outcomes, they assist couples in evaluating reproductive risks, comprehending the implications of their genetic status, and exploring their options. A thorough fertility treatment plan must include genetic counseling to guarantee that patients are informed and supported during their reproductive journey.

The study of variations in gene expression that do not result from modifications to the underlying DNA sequence is known as epigenetics. Fertility can be affected by epigenetic alterations brought on by environmental variables, lifestyle decisions, and even stress. Epigenetics research reveals how these variables affect reproductive health and how counteracting measures can be created. By addressing not only genetic issues but also the larger context of an individual's environment and health, an understanding of epigenetic impacts enables more focused and successful reproductive therapies.

Advances in Technologies for Assisted Reproduction (ART)
Since the first IVF birth in 1978, assisted reproductive technologies (ART) have advanced significantly. By increasing success rates and

making treatments more widely available and efficient, advances in ART
have increased the options available to infertile people and couples.
The mainstay of ART is still in vitro fertilization (IVF), which has seen
several advancements that have increased its effectiveness. One such
invention is time-lapse imaging, which enables embryologists to
continuously track the development of embryos without disturbing them.
The most viable embryos for transfer can be chosen with the use of this
technique, which offers comprehensive information about embryo
growth patterns. IVF success has also been increased by improvements
in embryo quality and implantation rates brought about by advancements
in culture media and laboratory techniques.

To aid in conception, intracytoplasmic sperm injection, or ICSI, entails
inserting a single sperm straight into an egg. For those with severe male
factor infertility, such as low sperm count or poor sperm motility, this
method is especially helpful. The success rates of IVF for couples
dealing with male infertility concerns have significantly increased
because of ICSI. Moreover, to guarantee that only healthy embryos are
transplanted, ICSI can be performed in tandem with genetic testing.
Donating eggs and sperm has increased the number of reproductive
choices available to people and couples who are unable to conceive with
their gametes. Donor-assisted ART success rates have increased because
of advancements in donor screening and matching. Donating eggs and
sperm has given same-sex couples, single parents, and people with
genetic disorders that affect their fertility new hope. Strict screening
procedures provide the best donor gametes, which raises the possibility
of positive results.

Using a gestational carrier to carry a pregnancy for people or couples who are unable to do it themselves is known as surrogacy. The success rates of surrogacy have increased due to developments in IVF and embryo transfer methods. In surrogacy agreements, legal and ethical issues are crucial since they guarantee the protection of each party's rights and welfare. For same-sex male couples, those with medical disorders that prohibit pregnancy, and people who have had surgery on their reproductive organs, surrogacy has emerged as a feasible option.

Fertility Preservation: For patients undergoing medical procedures that could affect their reproductive health, fertility preservation is now a feasible alternative thanks to developments in cryopreservation technology. Freezing eggs, sperm, and embryos enables people to maintain their fertility for later use. For cancer patients receiving radiation or chemotherapy, this technique has proven especially helpful.

By providing flexibility and optimism, fertility preservation empowers people to confidently manage their reproductive destiny.

Reproductive medicine is changing as a result of artificial intelligence (AI) and machine learning, which improve data analysis and decision-making. AI-powered technologies can determine which embryos are the most viable, forecast ART success rates, and customize treatment regimens. For instance, AI is used by embryo grading algorithms to evaluate the quality of embryos according to developmental and morphological standards. With the aid of these tools, doctors may better treat patients individually, increase success rates, and optimize fertility therapies.

Stem Cell Therapy: This new discipline has the potential to completely transform fertility treatments. The use of stem cells to repair ovarian tissue, enhance the quality of eggs, and increase fertility in women with reduced ovarian reserve or premature ovarian failure is still being investigated. Additionally, by enhancing sperm production and rebuilding testicular tissue, stem cell therapy shows promise in treating male infertility. Even though it is still in the experimental phase, stem cell therapy presents intriguing prospects for reproductive health in the future.

Non-Invasive Prenatal Testing (NIPT): NIPT is a state-of-the-art procedure that checks for genetic abnormalities by analyzing cell-free fetal DNA in a pregnant woman's blood. Without the dangers of invasive treatments like amniocentesis, this non-invasive test offers important information about the fetus's health. Trisomy 18, trisomy 13, and Down syndrome are among the diseases that NIPT may accurately identify. Prenatal care has been transformed by the availability of NIPT, which provides expectant parents with early detection of possible problems and peace of mind.

Gene editing: Genetic abnormalities that result in infertility or other genetic problems may be corrected by gene editing technologies like CRISPR-Cas9. Although it is currently in the early stage, gene editing presents the potential to treat the underlying genetic reasons for infertility. To guarantee the safe and responsible use of gene editing technologies, ethical considerations, and regulatory frameworks are crucial during development and implementation.

Microfluidics and Lab-on-a-Chip Technologies: These cutting-edge instruments simplify and improve several ART-related processes. These technologies use microchips to manipulate tiny fluid amounts to carry out intricate laboratory procedures. Microfluidics can be applied to genetic testing, embryo culture, and sperm sorting in reproductive medicine. Lab-on-a-chip technologies increase the efficacy and efficiency of reproductive treatments by providing greater precision, lower prices, and quicker outcomes.

In conclusion, the field of fertility treatment has changed as a result of advancements in assisted reproductive technology and genetic testing. These developments open up new opportunities.

Chapter 4: The Significance of Diet and Lifestyle

Because dietary and lifestyle decisions can have a substantial impact on reproductive health, research on the relationship between nutrition lifestyle, and fertility is vital. A comprehensive strategy for enhancing reproductive outcomes must include evidence-based nutritional recommendations, consistent exercise, and efficient stress management. We will go into great detail about these topics in this chapter, offering advice on how individuals and couples can make the best decisions for their reproductive health.

Evidence-Based Fertility Dietary Guidelines
A healthy, well-balanced diet is essential for preserving fertility and general health. Certain nutrients and dietary habits have been found to increase fertility in both men and women. The following food suggestions are supported by research and can increase fertility:

1. Healthy Fats: Research has linked increased fertility to the consumption of healthy fats, especially omega-3 fatty acids. Flaxseeds, chia seeds, walnuts, and fatty fish (including salmon, mackerel, and sardines) are foods high in omega-3 fatty acids. These fats promote reproductive health and lessen inflammation.

2. *Whole Grains:* Whole grains are a great way to get vitamins, minerals, and fiber. They support general health and aid in blood sugar regulation. Fertility can be enhanced by including whole grains in the diet, such as brown rice, quinoa, oats, and whole wheat.

3. *Vegetables and Fruits:* A diet high in fruits and vegetables offers vital antioxidants, vitamins, and minerals. The health of the reproductive system depends on these nutrients. For a well-rounded nutrient intake, try to incorporate a range of vibrant fruits and vegetables into your regular meals.

4. *Lean Proteins:* For general health and fertility, lean proteins—like those found in fish, poultry, turkey, beans, and legumes—are crucial. The synthesis of hormones as well as tissue upkeep and repair depend on protein.

5. *Dairy and Substitutes:* Calcium and vitamin D can be found in dairy products and their substitutes, such as fortified plant-based milk. A balanced diet should contain these nutrients since they are important for reproductive health.

6. *Hydration:* Maintaining proper hydration is essential for both fertility and general wellness. To support body processes and preserve optimum health, make it a point to sip on lots of water throughout the day.

7. *Reduce Sugar and Processed Foods:* Sugary drinks and processed foods might have a detrimental effect on fertility. These foods frequently contain a lot of added sugars, bad fats, and artificial chemicals, all of which can lead to hormone imbalances and inflammation. Reproductive health can be supported by consuming fewer of these foods.

8. *Moderate Alcohol Use:* Drinking too much alcohol can have a detrimental effect on fertility. Moderate alcohol consumption is advised since excessive alcohol can interfere with hormone balance and reproductive function.

9. *Steer clear of trans fats:* These fats, which are included in fried and processed meals, have been related to poor fertility outcomes. Reproductive health can be supported by avoiding trans fats and choosing healthy fats instead.

10. *Supplements:* To promote fertility, supplements may occasionally be suggested. For women who are trying to conceive, folic acid, vitamin B12, and omega-3 supplements are frequently recommended. Before beginning any supplements, it is crucial to speak with a healthcare professional to be sure they are suitable for your needs.

Exercise and Fertility: Advantages and Recommendations
Another essential element of a healthy lifestyle that can have a good effect on fertility is regular physical activity. Numerous advantages of exercise include stress reduction, weight management, and enhanced

cardiovascular health. The following rules can help you incorporate exercise into a lifestyle that promotes fertility:

1. Aerobic Exercise: Walking, jogging, cycling, and swimming are examples of aerobic workouts that can enhance general fitness and promote reproductive health. Every week, try to get in at least 150 minutes of moderate-intensity aerobic activity.

2. Strength Training: Including strength training activities, like bodyweight or weightlifting, can enhance metabolic health and aid in muscle growth. Every week, try to get in at least two days of weight exercise.

3. Flexibility and Balance: Exercises like yoga and pilates that enhance these qualities help lower stress and enhance general well-being. Additionally, these workouts can enhance reproductive health and reduce menstrual pain.

4. Steer clear of Overexertion: Although regular exercise has many advantages, excessive exercise might impair fertility. Particularly if you are attempting to conceive, it is crucial to pay attention to your body and refrain from engaging in excessive or strenuous exercise.

5. Remain Consistent: When it comes to working out, consistency is essential. Long-term advantages for reproductive health can result from establishing and maintaining a regular fitness regimen.

Stress Management and Its Effect on Reproductive Health

Stress can significantly impair reproductive function and hormonal balance, which in turn can affect fertility. Optimizing fertility results requires appropriate stress management. The following are some methods for reducing stress and enhancing reproductive health:

1. Mindfulness and Meditation: These techniques can help lower stress and enhance general well-being. These methods can improve reproductive health and encourage calm.

2. Counseling and Support: Joining support groups or seeking counseling can help manage stress and offer emotional support. It can be helpful to speak with an expert or make connections with people who are experiencing similar things.

3. Healthy Coping Strategies: Stress can be decreased by using healthy coping strategies like hobbies, social interactions, and relaxation techniques. Choose enjoyable and soothing hobbies and include them in your daily schedule.

4. Adequate Sleep: Stress reduction and general health depend on getting adequate sleep. To promote hormonal balance and reproductive health, try to get between seven and nine hours of good sleep each night.

5. Time Management: Productivity may be increased and stress can be decreased with good time management. To prevent feeling overburdened, prioritize your responsibilities, establish reasonable goals, and make a balanced timetable.

6. *Healthy ties:* Keeping up good ties with spouses, family, and friends helps ease stress and offer emotional support. Stress management and reproductive health promotion require open communication and reciprocal support.

In summary, dietary and lifestyle factors have a complex and crucial impact on fertility and reproductive health. Individuals and couples can improve their overall well-being and reproductive results by adhering to evidence-based dietary recommendations, exercising frequently, and effectively managing stress. To create individualized programs that take into account each patient's needs and objectives, it is crucial to confer with healthcare professionals.

Section Three

Comprehensive Fertility Care

Chapter 5: Alternative and Natural Medicines

Being a parent can be an extremely personal and frequently difficult experience. Many people and couples use natural and alternative therapies to supplement conventional medical treatments, even though modern science has made great progress in understanding and treating reproductive concerns. These holistic methods seek to promote general well-being and improve reproductive health by highlighting the connection between the mind, body, and spirit. Acupuncture, herbal medicine, mindfulness, meditation, yoga, and the function of holistic practitioners in reproductive care are just a few of the natural and alternative therapies that we will examine in this chapter.

Herbal Medicine, Acupuncture, and Other Natural Therapies

The use of acupuncture
Thin needles are inserted into particular body spots during acupuncture, an ancient Chinese medical procedure, to encourage the passage of energy and aid in healing. For thousands of years, it has been used to cure a wide range of illnesses, including infertility. Numerous studies have demonstrated the potential advantages of acupuncture, which has become more and more popular in recent years as a supplemental treatment for infertility problems.

The Operation of Acupuncture
The vital energy known as "qi" travels through the body along the meridians, according to traditional Chinese medicine (TCM). A disturbance in the flow of qi can result in imbalances and sickness. By activating particular places on the body called acupoints, acupuncture seeks to restore the equilibrium of qi, encourage the flow of energy, and improve general health.

Acupuncture is thought to increase blood flow to the reproductive organs, balance hormones, lessen stress, and improve the reproductive system's general performance of fertility. Sessions may be held weekly or as advised by the practitioner, and acupuncture treatments are usually tailored to the individual's unique needs and conditions.

Studies on Fertility and Acupuncture

Numerous research have looked into how acupuncture affects fertility, especially in women receiving in vitro fertilization (IVF) or other assisted reproductive technologies (ART). Acupuncture has been proven to increase follicle count, enhance implantation rates, and increase endometrial thickness, all of which may improve IVF outcomes. Acupuncture has also been linked to lower levels of stress and anxiety, which may have a beneficial effect on reproductive health. A lot of people and couples find acupuncture to be a helpful and encouraging treatment on their fertility journey, even if more research is required to completely understand the processes and efficacy of this treatment.

Herbal Remedies

Another essential element of traditional Chinese medicine and other traditional healing systems is herbal medicine. It entails the application of plant-based treatments to promote general health and treat particular medical issues. For millennia, people have utilized herbal therapy to improve reproductive health and increase fertility.

Frequently Used Fertility Herbs

Known as the "female ginseng," dong quai (Angelica sinensis) is frequently used to restore hormonal balance, enhance blood flow to the reproductive organs, and control menstrual cycles.

The chaste tree, or Vitex agnus-castus, is used to support the production of progesterone, a hormone necessary to sustain pregnancy and control menstrual cycles.

The phytoestrogens found in red clover (Trifolium pratense) can help balance estrogen levels and promote reproductive health.

Maca root (Lepidium meyenii): Known for its adaptogenic qualities, maca is believed to boost libido, promote hormonal balance, and improve general vigor.

The adaptogenic herb ashwagandha (Withania somnifera) promotes hormonal balance, lowers stress, and enhances reproductive health in general. The raspberry leaf (Rubus idaeus) is frequently used to promote reproductive health and tone the uterus. In order to prepare for childbirth and strengthen the uterus, it is frequently advised throughout pregnancy.

Studies on Fertility and Herbal Medicine

The use of herbal therapy for fertility is supported by a plethora of traditional knowledge, although there is currently little empirical evidence of its efficacy. Although some research has indicated that some herbs are beneficial for reproductive health, more thorough clinical trials are required to determine their safety and effectiveness. Before utilizing herbal remedies, people should speak with a certified healthcare professional because they may not be appropriate for everyone and can interfere with pharmaceuticals.

Additional Natural Remedies

To enhance fertility, several additional natural therapies are frequently employed in addition to acupuncture and herbal medicine:

Reproductive health can be supported by a well-balanced diet full of vital minerals like folic acid, iron, zinc, and omega-3 fatty acids. To improve fertility and correct particular deficits, supplements could be suggested.

Enhancing blood flow to the reproductive organs, lowering stress levels, and encouraging relaxation are the main goals of fertility massage therapy. Reflexology and belly massage are two methods that can be used to promote reproductive health.

The use of water for therapeutic purposes is known as hydrotherapy. Methods like contrast showers, sitz baths, and heated baths help enhance circulation, encourage relaxation, and enhance general well-being.

Yoga, Meditation, and Mindfulness for Fertility
Meditation and Mindfulness

Practices like mindfulness and meditation entail concentrating on the here and now while developing an attitude of acceptance and awareness. Because of their capacity to lower stress, promote emotional stability, and boost general health, these techniques have grown in popularity.

The Advantages of Meditation and Mindfulness for Fertility

The menstrual cycle and hormonal balance can be upset by stress and anxiety, which can have a major effect on reproductive health. Stress reduction and relaxation are two benefits of mindfulness and meditation that may enhance reproductive results. In addition to improving emotional resilience, mindfulness and meditation practices can assist people in managing the difficulties and unknowns associated with the fertility process.

Methods for Meditation and Mindfulness Practice

- Mindful Breathing: Concentrate on your breath and notice how it feels to inhale and exhale. This technique encourages relaxation and helps focus attention on the here and now.

Body Scan Meditation: Pay attention to various body parts and note any tension or discomfort. Relaxation and a sense of physical connectedness are encouraged by this technique.

- Loving-Kindness Meditation: Develop kindness and compassion for both yourself and other people. This technique helps lessen stress and improve emotional health.

Guided Visualization: Construct positive mental images by using visualization and imagery, such as picturing a successful conception and a healthy pregnancy. This technique helps lessen anxiety and encourage a positive outlook.

Fertility Yoga

Yoga is an age-old discipline that enhances mental, emotional, and spiritual health by combining physical postures, breathwork, and meditation. Numerous health advantages of yoga have been demonstrated, such as stress reduction, increased flexibility, and improved general health.

Yoga's Advantages for Fertility

For both individuals and couples attempting to conceive, yoga can be a beneficial exercise. The asanas, or physical postures, increase flexibility, encourage relaxation, and improve blood flow to the reproductive organs. Yoga's breathwork and meditation techniques can help people feel less stressed and anxious while promoting reproductive health and hormonal balance.

Yoga Pose for Getting Pregnant
Bound Angle position (Baddha Konasana): This position increases blood flow to the pelvic area by opening the hips. Additionally, it eases tension and encourages relaxation.

- Viparita Karani's Legs Up the Wall Pose: This healing pose encourages relaxation, lowers stress, and improves circulation. It is frequently advised to increase the likelihood of conception after sexual activity.

The bridge posture, also known as setu bandhasana, increases blood flow to the reproductive organs, relaxes the body, and strengthens the pelvic floor muscles.

The Cat-Cow Pose (Marjaryasana-Bitilasana) is a smooth transition between two positions that helps ease tension, increase relaxation, and enhance spinal flexibility.

- Child's position (Balasana): This calming position eases tension, encourages relaxation, and gently extends the hips and lower back.

Mind-Body Fertility Techniques
Yoga, mindfulness, meditation, and other mind-body techniques can be effective means of promoting fertility and general health. By encouraging relaxation, lowering stress levels, and strengthening emotional fortitude, these techniques foster a favorable environment for conception.

The Function of Holistic Medical Professionals in Fertility Treatment

When it comes to helping individuals and couples in their reproductive journey, holistic practitioners are essential. By treating the mental, emotional, and spiritual facets of reproductive health, these professionals take a holistic approach to fertility care. Some important roles that holistic practitioners may play in fertility care include the following:

Practitioners of Integrative Medicine

Practitioners of integrative medicine offer a comprehensive approach to reproductive care by combining evidence-based complementary therapies with traditional medical treatments. Physicians who practice integrative medicine, naturopathy, and holistic health may be among these professionals. They collaborate with patients to create individualized treatment programs that cater to their particular requirements and objectives.

Practitioners of Acupuncture

Professionals with training in acupuncture and other facets of traditional Chinese medicine are known as acupuncturists. They determine the health and fertility status of their patients, spot energy flow abnormalities in the body, and create individualized therapy regimens. To promote reproductive health, acupuncturists may also offer nutrition and lifestyle advice.

Herbalists

Practitioners who focus on using plant-based medicines to promote health and well-being are known as herbalists. They evaluate the medical conditions of their patients, suggest particular herbs and formulations, and offer advice on how to utilize herbal medicine safely and effectively. To guarantee a thorough approach to reproductive therapy, herbalists may also collaborate with other medical professionals.

Teachers of Yoga

Fertility-focused yoga instructors offer advice on breathing techniques, yoga positions, and meditation techniques that promote reproductive health. To meet the requirements of single people and couples attempting to conceive, they might provide solo sessions or group classes. Yoga teachers can contribute to the development of a caring and encouraging atmosphere for yoga and mind-body practices.

Dietitians and nutritionists

Professionals with expertise in the science of nutrition and how it affects health include dietitians and nutritionists. By offering individualized nutrition programs and evidence-based dietary recommendations to enhance reproductive health, they play a crucial role in fertility care. They contribute in the following ways:

Individualized Dietary Programs

Dietitians and nutritionists evaluate the nutritional health of individuals and couples attempting to conceive, taking into account lifestyle, dietary preferences, medical history, and age. They create individualized diet programs that maximize hormonal balance, correct certain nutrient deficits, and improve fertility in general. Meal planning, dietary supplements, and suggestions for macronutrient and micronutrient intake may all be included in these plans.

Guidance for Education

Dietitians and nutritionists offer instructional advice on the value of a well-balanced diet and how it affects reproductive health. They provide helpful guidance on choosing nutritious foods, avoiding dietary hazards that may impair fertility, and adding nutrient-rich foods to regular meals. Topics include quantity control, cooking methods to maintain nutrient content, and the advantages of particular nutrients may be covered in educational sessions.

Assistance with Special Dietary Requirements

Specialized nutritional care may be necessary for those with particular dietary demands, such as those who have food allergies, intolerances, or long-term medical disorders. Dietitians and nutritionists collaborate with these people to create safe and efficient eating plans that meet their specific nutritional requirements and promote fertility. For instance, they might offer advice on low-glycemic index meals for people with PCOS, gluten- or dairy-free diets, or anti-inflammatory diets for people with endometriosis.

Behavioral and Lifestyle Counseling

Nutritionists and dietitians provide lifestyle and behavioral counseling in addition to dietary recommendations to promote reproductive health and general well-being. This could involve advice on how to keep a healthy weight, develop good eating habits, and manage stress through mindful eating. They assist individuals and couples in creating a conducive environment for conception by addressing lifestyle issues that impact fertility.

An Integrated Method for Fertility Treatment

A thorough and all-encompassing approach to reproductive care is provided by combining traditional medical treatments with complementary and alternative therapies. By empowering individuals and couples to take control of their fertility journey, this integrative approach acknowledges the significance of addressing the physical, mental, and spiritual elements of reproductive health.

Cooperative Healthcare

A multidisciplinary team of medical professionals, such as reproductive endocrinologists, integrative medicine specialists, acupuncturists, herbalists, dietitians, yoga teachers, and mental health specialists, frequently collaborates to provide holistic fertility care. Together, these professionals can create thorough, individualized therapy programs that cater to the particular requirements and objectives of every person or couple.

Tailored Therapy Programs

Each person or couple's unique fertility issues and medical factors are taken into account while creating a personalized treatment plan. In addition to natural and alternative therapies like acupuncture, herbal medicine, mindfulness exercises, and diet, these strategies might combine medical treatments like hormonal therapies and assisted reproductive technology (ART). The objective is to establish a caring and encouraging atmosphere that improves reproductive health and raises the likelihood of a successful conception.

Empowerment of Patients

By giving people and couples the information and resources they need to make educated decisions about their reproductive health, a holistic approach to fertility treatment empowers them. This includes advice on natural and alternative therapies, education on how nutrition and lifestyle choices affect fertility, and assistance with mental and emotional health. Individuals and couples can increase their chances of a successful pregnancy and enhance their general health by actively participating in their reproductive journey.

Mental and Emotional Health

An essential part of reproductive care is the mental and emotional health of both individuals and couples. Taking care of one's mental health is crucial for general well-being because the reproductive process can be emotionally taxing. Yoga, meditation, mindfulness, and counseling are all used in holistic fertility therapy to promote emotional resilience and lower stress levels. These techniques give people and couples more confidence and relaxation as they deal with the difficulties of infertility.

Relationship Between Mind and Body

A key tenet of holistic fertility therapy is the mind-body link. Given that stress, anxiety, and negative emotions can affect reproductive health, this connection highlights the interaction between mental, emotional, and physical health. Mind-body techniques can improve fertility outcomes and reproductive health by encouraging relaxation, lowering stress, and cultivating a positive outlook.

Spiritual Assistance

Another crucial component of holistic fertility care is spiritual assistance. During the fertility process, faith offers many people and couples a feeling of direction, optimism, and connection. Prayer, meditation, and time spent in nature are examples of spiritual activities that can offer emotional support as well as promote acceptance and serenity. Finding purpose and resiliency in the face of fertility difficulties can also be facilitated by spiritual assistance for people and couples.

In summary, a variety of natural and alternative therapies that promote the mind, body, and spirit are included in holistic care for fertility. To improve reproductive health and assist individuals and couples on their fertility journey, holistic practitioners' advice, acupuncture, herbal medicine, yoga, and mindfulness exercises are essential. Holistic fertility care is a thorough and individualized strategy that enables people to maximize their reproductive health and raise their chances of a successful pregnancy by combining these therapies with traditional medical treatments. We are getting closer to establishing a kind and encouraging atmosphere for everyone looking to start a family as we investigate and adopt more holistic approaches to fertility.

Chapter 6: Psychological and Emotional Assistance

The parenting path is frequently a time of excitement and expectation, but it may also be a time of emotional and psychological difficulties for many infertile individuals and couples. Many other feelings, including despair, frustration, guilt, and anxiety, can be triggered by infertility. Maintaining mental health and well-being requires overcoming these emotional obstacles. This chapter will cover several techniques for coping with the psychological effects of infertility, the value of support networks and available counseling, and methods for fostering resilience and preserving hope along the path.

Managing the Emotional Difficulties of Infertility
For both individuals and couples, infertility is a very personal and frequently upsetting process that may be emotionally taxing. A variety of emotional reactions may result from the inability to conceive as well as the ambiguity surrounding the results of treatment. The first step in managing the difficulties of infertility is to recognize and understand these feelings.

Typical Feelings in Reaction to Infertility

Grief and Loss: When a person or couple is unable to conceive, they often feel a sense of loss and grief. The loss of the desired future, the loss of bodily control, and the loss of the chance to have children can all be linked to this grief. It's critical to understand that these grief-related emotions are real and deserving of recognition.

Anger and Frustration: Being infertile can be an upsetting experience, particularly if medical interventions don't produce the expected outcomes. Feelings of injustice or the belief that one's body is betraying them can also cause anger. It's critical to control and healthily express your rage.

Shame and Guilt: A lot of people and couples experience shame or guilt due to their infertility. They can feel inadequate in some way or blame themselves. The expectations and pressures placed on parents by society might make these emotions worse. It's critical to combat these pessimistic ideas and understand that infertility does not indicate one's value.

Anxiety and Worry: These emotions might be brought on by the uncertainty surrounding infertility treatments as well as a dread of the unknown. Anxiety can be increased by worries about financial expenses, the negative effects of treatments, and the effect on one's relationship. Maintaining mental health requires learning anxiety management techniques.

Depression and loneliness: Feelings of depression and loneliness can result from the emotional strain of infertility. People and couples may avoid interacting with friends and family who have children or retreat from social events. Emotional well-being depends on identifying the symptoms of depression and getting help.

Techniques for Handling Emotional Difficulties

Recognize and Validate Emotions: It's critical to recognize and validate the feelings connected to infertility. Give yourself permission to experience and communicate these feelings without passing judgment. Talking to a therapist, partner, or trusted friend about your feelings can help you feel better. Develop self-compassion by treating oneself with kindness and compassion. Acknowledge that you are trying your hardest to cope with the difficult experience of infertility. Take care of yourself and do things that make you happy and calm you down.

Establish Reasonable Expectations: Having reasonable expectations regarding the fertility process will help you deal with frustration and disappointment. Recognize that not every cycle will result in a pregnancy and that fertility treatments may take some time. Take things one step at a time and acknowledge minor accomplishments as you go.

Create Healthy Coping Mechanisms: Look for constructive strategies to deal with stress and unpleasant feelings. This could be taking up hobbies, working out, keeping a journal, or meditating and being attentive. Steer clear of unhealthy coping strategies like substance abuse or over-avoidance.

Open Communication with Your Partner: Relationships may suffer as a result of infertility. Maintaining a solid and encouraging relationship with your partner requires open and honest communication.

Communicate your emotions, talk about your worries, and cooperate to overcome the obstacles posed by infertility.

Seek expert Support: To cope with the emotional difficulties of infertility, seeking help from a mental health expert, such as a therapist or counselor, can be very beneficial. Therapy can provide a secure environment for you to examine your feelings, create coping mechanisms, and strengthen your resilience.

Options for Counseling and Support Networks

Having a solid support network is essential for coping with the psychological effects of infertility. Numerous people can offer help, such as friends, family, support groups, and licensed counselors. Throughout their fertility journey, individuals and couples can feel less alone and more powerful by getting the right assistance.

Systems of Support

Support from Your Partner: Throughout the fertility process, your partner may be your main source of assistance. Navigating the difficulties together requires you to keep lines of communication open and strengthen your bond. Take part in activities that promote intimacy and connection while providing each other with practical and emotional assistance.

Family and Friends: Reliable family members and friends can offer consolation and emotional support. Talking to loved ones about your feelings and experiences might make you feel less alone and more connected to the community. To make sure the support you receive is beneficial and considerate, it's critical to establish boundaries and express your needs.

Support Groups: Participating in a support group for infertile individuals and couples can help one feel understood and like they belong. Support groups provide a forum for people facing comparable difficulties to exchange stories, acquire new perspectives, and offer support. Meetings in person and participating in online forums can both be excellent means of fostering connections.

Community and Faith-Based groups: For infertile people and couples, community and faith-based groups may provide support services. These associations can offer tools, support groups, and therapy to assist deal with the psychological and practical effects of infertility.

Options for Counseling

Individual therapy: Individual therapy offers a therapeutic environment where you can work on personal development, explore your feelings, and create coping mechanisms one-on-one. A qualified therapist can assist you in managing stress and anxiety as well as specific infertility-related issues.

Couples Counseling: The goal of couples counseling is to improve the bond between partners and deal with the effects of infertility on the partnership. A qualified therapist can assist in enhancing mutual support, resolving disputes, and improving communication. Counseling for couples can be especially helpful when it comes to managing emotional difficulties and making decisions regarding reproductive treatments.

Group Therapy: In group therapy, a small group of people meet with a therapist on a regular basis to talk about their experiences and offer support to one another. As participants discuss their challenges and triumphs, group therapy can provide a sense of belonging and validation. People who are looking for understanding and connection from others going through similar struggles may find this therapeutic approach particularly beneficial.

The goal of mind-body therapy is to enhance general well-being by combining psychological and physical methods. Stress reduction, emotional resilience, and reproductive health are all supported by methods including mindfulness, meditation, yoga, and relaxation exercises. Counseling sessions, whether individual or group, can include mind-body therapy. Working with a qualified coach who specializes in fertility concerns is known as fertility coaching. Throughout the process of becoming pregnant, fertility coaches offer individualized assistance, direction, and knowledge. They assist individuals and couples in navigating medical treatments, making well-informed decisions, and creating coping mechanisms for emotions and stress.
Increasing Resilience and Preserving Hope

The road to infertility can be emotionally and psychologically taxing, frequently marked by dejection, frustration, and pessimism. Navigating these obstacles and finding the strength to proceed on the parenting journey requires developing resilience and holding onto hope. Hope is the conviction that good things are achievable, while resilience is the capacity to adjust and flourish in the face of hardship. They work well together to help people and couples deal with the psychological effects of infertility.

Resilience on an emotional level

Developing coping skills and techniques to control stress, adjust to change, and overcome setbacks is a key component of emotional resilience. The following are some essential techniques for developing emotional fortitude throughout the process of becoming pregnant:

1. Self-Compassion: Self-compassion entails treating oneself with kindness and understanding, particularly when things are tough. It entails accepting the suffering and annoyance of infertility without passing judgment or feeling guilty about it. Self-compassionate people can treat themselves with the same consideration and consideration that they would a friend.

2. Acceptance and Mindfulness: Mindfulness is focusing on the here and now without passing judgment. By practicing mindfulness, people can avoid worrying about the past or the future and instead remain centered and grounded in the here and now. Recognizing and accepting the situation as it is, despite its difficulty, is the essence of acceptance. Acceptance and mindfulness work together to lower stress and enhance emotional health.

3. Positive Reframing: This technique entails taking a fresh look at a situation and seeing its advantages or room for development. Finding methods to see the difficulties and suffering more positively is preferable to ignoring them. For instance, people can recognize the work they did and the knowledge they acquired rather than dwelling on the frustration of a treatment that didn't work.

4. *Creating a Support System:* Emotional resilience depends on having a solid support system of friends, family, and medical professionals. others can feel less alone and receive emotional relief by talking to trusted others about their experiences and feelings. Online and in-person support groups can also provide beneficial contacts with those experiencing similar things.

5. Having reasonable expectations means being aware that the reproductive process may be rocky at times and that it might take some time to get the results you want. People can lessen the strain and stress related to the fertility process by regulating expectations and establishing realistic goals.

6. *Taking Care of Oneself:* Self-care entails setting aside time to take care of one's physical, emotional, and mental needs. Exercise, hobbies, relaxation methods, and spending time with loved ones are a few examples of this. Making self-care a priority enables people to refuel and preserve their emotional fortitude.

Keeping Hope Alive

Sustaining optimism and motivation throughout the reproductive process requires holding onto hope. Even in the face of obstacles, hope can give you the willpower and perseverance to keep going. The following techniques can help you stay hopeful:

1. *Creating Positive Intentions:* Creating positive intentions entails concentrating on one's goals and imagining successful outcomes. This can give people a feeling of direction and purpose, which keeps them inspired and upbeat. These goals can be strengthened and a positive outlook encouraged by using visualization techniques and positive affirmations.

2. Honoring Little Victories: Honoring minor victories and significant junctures during the conception process may keep spirits high and a sense of advancement alive. A sense of hope and accomplishment can be fostered by recognizing and enjoying these accomplishments, whether they include finishing a treatment cycle, getting positive test results, or obtaining emotional support.

3. Looking for Inspirational Stories: It can be encouraging and motivating to read or hear about the stories of those who have surmounted infertility obstacles. Inspirational tales of tenacity, perseverance, and successful pregnancies can inspire optimism. These tales serve as a reminder to people that they are not alone and that good things can happen.

4. Keeping the Bigger Picture in Mind: Keeping the big picture in mind entails keeping the end aim in mind and maintaining perspective. It entails realizing that there are numerous other facets of life to treasure and savor and that the fertility journey is only one of them. People can keep a sense of balance and hope by keeping their eyes on the wider picture.

5. *Examining Alternative Routes to Parenthood:* For individuals dealing with severe infertility issues, investigating alternate routes to parenthood, such as adoption or surrogacy, might offer options and hope. The knowledge that there are various approaches to starting a family might provide comfort and optimism for the future.

6. *Developing a Spiritual Connection:* For many people, spirituality is a source of strength, consolation, and hope. Spirituality, whether via meditation, religious activities, or a relationship with nature, can provide comfort and hope in trying times. People can discover meaning and purpose in their journeys by engaging in spiritual practices.

Expert Assistance

Building resilience and preserving hope can be greatly aided by seeking professional assistance from mental health specialists, such as therapists and counselors. Therapy can offer a secure setting for processing feelings, creating coping mechanisms, and investigating methods to maintain hope. The emotional and psychological difficulties of infertility can be successfully addressed by a variety of therapeutic modalities, including solution-focused therapy, mindfulness-based therapy, and cognitive-behavioral therapy (CBT).

Couples Counseling

During the fertility process, couples can benefit from therapy to increase communication and fortify their bond. Couples therapy offers an environment for sharing experiences, expressing feelings, and offering support to one another. It can also strengthen a couple's sense of unity and partnership as they go through the difficulties and stress of infertility together.

Programs for the Mind and Body

Mind-body therapies created especially for infertile individuals and couples can provide all-encompassing emotional and psychological assistance. To address the particular difficulties of the reproductive journey, these programs frequently incorporate aspects of yoga, meditation, mindfulness, and cognitive-behavioral approaches. Participants can connect with others in similar circumstances, acquire useful coping mechanisms, and lessen stress.

In conclusion, overcoming the psychological and emotional obstacles of infertility requires fostering resilience and preserving optimism. Self-compassion, mindfulness, positive reframing, and self-care are practices that help people become emotionally resilient and adjust to the highs and lows of the fertility process. The courage and inspiration required to keep going can be found by keeping optimism alive through good intentions, acknowledging minor victories, and reading motivational tales. Therapy and mind-body programs are examples of professional support that can provide helpful techniques and resources for emotional regulation and maintaining hope. In the end, a comprehensive strategy that takes into account the mind, body, and spirit can enable people and couples to find hope, strength, and resilience as they prepare to become parents.

Section 4:

All-Inclusive Fertility Techniques

Chapter 7: Tailored Plans for Fertility

To address the particular requirements and situations of people and couples attempting to conceive, customized fertility programs are crucial. These plans entail developing customized approaches that take into account several variables, including age, medical history, lifestyle, and particular fertility issues. People can maximize their fertility and raise their chances of a successful pregnancy by creating a customized strategy. This chapter will cover how to design a customized fertility strategy, offer examples of effective customized fertility techniques, and go over the significance of collaborating with medical professionals to maximize fertility.

How to Design a Customized Fertility Strategy
Making a personalized fertility plan entails a thorough assessment of each person's unique situation and the creation of a unique strategy to deal with certain fertility issues. The following are essential steps for developing a customized fertility plan:

1. Comprehensive Evaluation: Having a complete evaluation by a medical professional is the first step in developing a customized fertility plan. To find any underlying reproductive problems, this evaluation may involve imaging scans, laboratory testing, physical examinations, and medical history. This may entail evaluating a woman's ovarian reserve, hormone levels, and reproductive organ health. Hormone testing and semen analysis may be part of it for men.

2. Determining Fertility Objectives: Following the evaluation, it's critical to determine precise fertility objectives. The desire to conceive naturally, with assisted reproductive technologies (ART), or through other means like adoption or surrogacy may fall under this category. Knowing these objectives aids in directing the creation of a customized plan.

3. Evaluating Lifestyle Factors: Fertility can be greatly impacted by lifestyle factors like nutrition, exercise, stress, and sleep. Optimizing reproductive health requires evaluating these variables and making the required modifications. This could entail putting an emphasis on getting enough sleep, controlling stress, eating a diet high in nutrients, and exercising frequently.

4. *Creating a Treatment Plan*: A treatment plan can be created based on the evaluation and goals that have been determined. In addition to natural and alternative therapies like acupuncture, herbal medicine, and mindfulness exercises, this strategy might involve medical treatments like hormone therapies or surgical procedures. To support general reproductive health and address particular fertility issues, the treatment plan should be customized.

5. *Tracking Progress:* To evaluate the success of the fertility plan and make the required modifications, routine tracking and follow-up are crucial. This could entail monitoring ovulation, menstrual cycles, and other reproductive indicators in addition to routine checkups with the doctor. Progress tracking keeps the plan in line with each person's requirements and objectives.

6. *Emotional and Psychological assistance:* An individualized fertility plan must include emotional and psychological assistance. Counseling, support groups, and mind-body techniques may be used to help with the emotional difficulties associated with infertility and to foster hope and resilience.

Examples of Effective Customized Fertility Techniques

Case Study 1: The Path to Parenthood for Sarah and John
For more than two years, Sarah and John had been unsuccessfully
attempting to conceive. Following a thorough assessment, it was
discovered that John had a low sperm count and Sarah had polycystic
ovarian syndrome (PCOS). A customized fertility plan comprising
medical treatments, alternative therapies, and lifestyle changes was
suggested by their healthcare physician.

A low-glycemic index diet, consistent exercise, and stress-reduction
methods like yoga and meditation were all part of Sarah's regimen. In
order to control her ovulation, she was also prescribed medication. It
was suggested that John take supplements to enhance the quality of his
sperm and reduce his exposure to environmental pollutants.

Along with these lifestyle adjustments, Sarah and John had acupuncture
sessions and intrauterine insemination (IUI) to lower stress and increase
blood flow to the reproductive organs. Nine months after undergoing
multiple IUI cycles, Sarah and John were able to conceive and welcome
their beautiful baby daughter. They achieved their intended result by
addressing lifestyle and medical concerns in their customized
reproductive plan.

Case Study 2: The Journey of Maria to Motherhood

Maria, a 38-year-old woman, was diagnosed with decreased ovarian reserve after suffering several miscarriages. To support her reproductive system and maximize her general health, her healthcare professional suggested a customized fertility strategy.

Maria's strategy called for regular exercise, stress-reduction techniques like mindfulness meditation, and a Mediterranean diet high in vitamins, antioxidants, and healthy fats. Additionally, she was prescribed drugs to strengthen the quality of her eggs and improve ovarian function.

Maria added natural medicines like red clover and coenzyme Q10 to her routine in addition to medical therapy. Additionally, preimplantation genetic testing (PGT) was used in conjunction with IVF to choose the healthiest embryos for transfer. Maria was able to conceive and give birth to a healthy boy despite the difficulties. Her success was largely attributed to her customized reproductive plan, which integrated lifestyle and alternative therapies with medical measures.

Case Study 3: The Surrogacy Journey of David and Lisa

After several unsuccessful IVF attempts, David and Lisa decided to look into surrogacy as a potential alternative to becoming parents. Their customized reproductive approach included creating a thorough surrogacy agreement and collaborating with a fertility clinic to identify a potential gestational carrier.

To guarantee the best quality embryos for transfer, David and Lisa underwent genetic testing and embryo screening. To deal with the psychological and legal ramifications of surrogacy, they also received guidance and assistance. Throughout the pregnancy, the gestational carrier received emotional and medical care.

Regular communication with the gestational carrier was part of David and Lisa's customized reproductive plan, which made sure that everyone involved was informed and encouraged. When their journey came to an end with the arrival of their twin sons, who were both healthy, they were thankful for the all-encompassing and customized approach that enabled them to fulfill their dream of becoming parents.

Cooperating with Medical Professionals to Increase Fertility
Working together with medical professionals is crucial to creating and carrying out customized fertility plans. Healthcare professionals assist individuals and couples on their fertility journey by contributing resources and knowledge. The following are crucial elements of collaborating with medical professionals to maximize fertility:

1. Open Communication: Creating a successful fertility plan requires candid and open communication with medical professionals. Patients and couples should discuss with their healthcare providers their medical history, lifestyle choices, and fertility objectives. Providers can use this information to customize the plan to fit individual needs.

2. *Multidisciplinary strategy:* A multidisciplinary strategy entails collaborating with a group of medical specialists, such as integrative medicine practitioners, acupuncturists, herbalists, nutritionists, reproductive endocrinologists, and mental health specialists. Comprehensive care that takes into account every facet of fertility and general health is ensured by this cooperative approach.

3. *Empowerment and Education:* Medical professionals are essential in informing individuals and couples about their options, methods, and treatments for conception. They enable patients to make knowledgeable decisions regarding their reproductive health by giving them evidence-based information. To actively participate in the reproductive journey, one must be empowered and educated.

4. *Personalized Care:* Personalized care entails adjusting methods and treatments to each person's or couple's particular requirements. Based on individual preferences, fertility objectives, and medical examinations, healthcare experts create personalized strategies. Personalized care promotes general health and increases the efficacy of reproductive therapies.

5. *Emotional Support:* Medical professionals provide support to address the psychological components of the journey since they understand the emotional difficulties associated with infertility. This could involve mind-body techniques, support groups, and counseling. Couples and individuals who receive emotional support are better able to handle stress, stay optimistic, and develop resilience.

6. *Continuous Monitoring and Adjustment*: To make sure fertility programs stay in line with each person's needs and objectives, they need to be continuously monitored and adjusted. Frequent medical examinations, follow-up consultations, and progress reports enable healthcare professionals to modify the strategy as needed. This dynamic strategy promotes overall reproductive health and increases the likelihood of success.

7. *Advocacy and Advocacy:* By organizing treatment, negotiating insurance coverage, and offering resources to aid in the fertility process, healthcare professionals act as advocates for their patients. Advocacy makes sure that people and couples have the help and tools they need to fulfill their reproductive objectives.

To sum up, customized fertility programs are crucial for maximizing reproductive health and raising the likelihood of a healthy pregnancy. Individuals and couples can address their particular reproductive issues and strive toward their goals by developing customized tactics. Successful individualized fertility strategy case studies emphasize the value of integrating lifestyle and alternative therapies with medical treatments. Because they offer tools, support, and experience throughout the process, collaborating with healthcare providers is essential to creating and carrying out successful fertility strategies. Individuals and couples can take control of their reproductive health and realize their aspirations of parenting with a thorough and individualized approach to fertility care.

Chapter 8: Integrating Holistic Care with Contemporary Science

A holistic approach to fertility that takes into account the mental, emotional, and spiritual facets of reproductive health is provided by the fusion of contemporary science and holistic medicine. Individuals and couples can increase their chances of conceiving successfully and preserving general health by combining medical therapies with holistic methods. This chapter will examine the advantages of combining medical and holistic therapies, present case examples of mixed approaches, and provide helpful advice for preserving a well-rounded approach to fertility care.

Combining Holistic Methods with Medical Treatments
Both holistic medicine and modern science have special advantages for fertility, and combining them can result in a more thorough and successful plan. The following are some essential guidelines for combining holistic methods with medical treatments:

1. Complementary Therapies: By treating underlying imbalances, lowering stress levels, and enhancing general health, holistic therapies including acupuncture, herbal medicine, and mind-body techniques can support medical treatments. These therapies can boost the body's natural healing processes and increase the efficacy of medical treatments.

2. Personalized Care: Creating individualized treatment programs that take into account the particular requirements and objectives of every person or couple is a key component of fusing contemporary science with holistic care. Together, healthcare professionals and holistic practitioners develop tailored plans that combine medical and holistic approaches.

3. Whole-Person Approach: The interdependence of the mind, body, and spirit is acknowledged in a whole-person approach to reproductive care. People can attain a more harmonic and balanced condition that promotes reproductive health by attending to their physical, emotional, and spiritual well-being.

4. Evidence-Based methods: Using evidence-based methods, which are backed by clinical experience and research, is essential to integrating contemporary science with holistic care. This guarantees that people receive therapies that are safe, efficient, and customized to meet their individual needs.

Examples of Combined Strategies

Case Study 1: The Holistic IVF Experience of Emily and Mark

After several unsuccessful efforts at natural conception, Emily and Mark, who had been attempting to conceive for more than three years, decided to explore IVF. To support the IVF process and increase their chances of success, their fertility physician suggested implementing holistic therapies.

Regular acupuncture sessions were part of Emily and Mark's customized fertility plan to lower stress and increase blood flow to the reproductive organs. To promote hormonal balance and egg quality, Emily also took herbal pills that were recommended by a traditional Chinese medicine (TCM) practitioner.

Emily and Mark used yoga and mindfulness meditation in addition to medical therapies to help them relax and manage stress. To improve their relationship and deal with the emotional difficulties of infertility, they underwent counseling.

Emily became pregnant after two IVF cycles, and she and Mark welcomed their healthy baby boy into the world. Their success was largely attributed to their combination of holistic therapies and medical treatments.

Case Study 2: Rachel's Comprehensive Strategy for Endometriosis Recovery

After receiving a diagnosis of endometriosis, Rachel experienced excruciating discomfort and difficulties conceiving. Her doctor suggested a thorough course of treatment that included both medical procedures and complementary therapies.

To relieve her problems and remove endometrial tissue, Rachel had laparoscopic surgery. After the procedure, she collaborated with a holistic practitioner to create a customized regimen that included herbal remedies, mind-body techniques, and dietary adjustments.

To lessen inflammation and promote general health, Rachel embraced an anti-inflammatory diet high in fruits, vegetables, and omega-3 fatty acids. To improve hormonal balance and manage discomfort, she used herbal supplements that included ginger and turmeric.

To cope with the psychological effects of endometriosis, Rachel went to a support group for women who had gone through similar things and engaged in mindfulness meditation. Her emotional health and stress management both improved as a result of these techniques.

Rachel's symptoms and general health have improved as a result of her integrative approach. She was able to conceive and give birth to a healthy baby girl after a few months.

Case Study 3: The Natural and Medical Fertility Plan of Tom and Lisa

For more than a year, Tom and Lisa had been unsuccessfully attempting to conceive. Lisa experienced irregular menstrual periods, and Tom was diagnosed with low sperm count. To address these conditions, their healthcare professional suggested a combination of medical treatments and holistic therapies.

Tom took medicine to increase the motility and production of sperm. He also included lifestyle modifications including consistent exercise, a diet high in nutrients, and stress-reduction methods.

Lisa took medicine to promote ovulation and control her menstrual cycle. Additionally, she collaborated with a holistic practitioner to create a strategy that includes herbal therapy, acupuncture, and dietary adjustments.

To reduce tension and encourage relaxation, Tom and Lisa engaged in yoga and mindfulness meditation. To improve their relationship and deal with the emotional difficulties of infertility, they also got counseling.

Following their combined plan for six months, Tom and Lisa were able to conceive and welcome their healthy baby boy. They achieved their intended result by addressing both the medical and holistic elements of fertility with a customized and integrative strategy.

Useful Advice for Preserving a Balanced Approach

To maintain a balanced approach to reproductive care, medical treatments, and holistic therapies must be integrated while maintaining general health. The following useful advice can help you adopt a balanced approach:

1. Work together with holistic practitioners and healthcare providers: Create a customized and thorough fertility plan in collaboration with a group of medical professionals and holistic practitioners. To make sure that all facets of health are taken care of, open communication and teamwork are crucial.

2. Establish Achievable Goals: For your fertility journey, establish attainable and reasonable goals. Recognize that there may be ups and downs in the process, and practice patience with your development. Realistic goal-setting lowers stress and keeps one's attitude upbeat.

3. Make Self-Care a Priority: Make self-care a priority by partaking in activities that enhance mental, emotional, and physical health. This includes relaxing methods, a healthy diet, frequent exercise, and enough sleep. Self-care promotes general health and resiliency.

4. Control Stress: Fertility can be significantly impacted by stress. Include stress-reduction methods in your everyday routine, such as yoga, meditation, mindfulness, and deep breathing exercises. By encouraging relaxation, these techniques lessen the detrimental effects of stress on reproductive health.

5. *Keep Up:* Keep up with the most recent developments in holistic therapies and reproductive treatments. Examine and comprehend your options, then talk to your healthcare providers about them. You can make decisions that are consistent with your values and goals when you are well-informed.

6. *Seek Support:* Ask friends, family, support groups, or counselors for emotional and psychological assistance. It can be consoling and lessening to share your feelings and experiences with others. Support systems are essential to emotional health.

7. *Have Flexibility:* If necessary, be willing to modify your fertility plan. Treatments may occasionally need to be adjusted in light of new knowledge or development. Being flexible enables you to adjust to changes and carry on with your reproductive quest.

8. *Pay Attention to the Big Picture:* Keep in mind that fertility is only one part of your life. Keep your eyes on the wider picture and find happiness in other aspects of your life, such as relationships, hobbies, and personal development. Keeping a balanced viewpoint keeps you resilient and optimistic.

In conclusion, a thorough and successful approach to fertility can be achieved by fusing contemporary research with holistic treatment. A well-rounded approach that takes into account the mental, emotional, and spiritual facets of reproductive health is offered by combining medical interventions with holistic therapies. The significance of individualized care and cooperation between healthcare professionals and holistic practitioners is demonstrated by case studies of effective combination tactics. Individuals and couples can maximize their fertility, improve their general well-being, and raise their chances of realizing their aspirations of motherhood by adhering to helpful advice for keeping a balanced attitude.

conclusion

Examining Fertility's Future

As we draw to a close this thorough examination of fertility, it is critical to take stock of the state of fertility treatments, future lines of inquiry, and possible discoveries that could benefit individuals and couples pursuing motherhood. Although the developments in holistic care and reproductive health offer a strong basis, there is still more room for creativity and empowerment in the future.

The Changing Fertility Treatment Landscape

Thanks to developments in medical research, technology, and our understanding of human reproduction, the field of fertility therapies is always changing. The future of fertility treatments is being shaped by several significant trends and advancements:

1. Precision Medicine: This field focuses on adjusting medical interventions to each patient's unique genetic, environmental, and lifestyle characteristics. Precision medicine seeks to provide individualized treatment regimens for fertility based on each patient's distinct genetic profile and reproductive health. This method lowers the possibility of unfavorable results while increasing the efficacy of therapies.

2. *Genetic and Genomic technology:* Fertility treatment is undergoing a revolution thanks to developments in genetic and genomic technology. Genetic variables that affect fertility may be found and addressed by methods including whole-genome sequencing, CRISPR gene editing, and epigenetic study. More precise diagnosis, focused treatments, and the avoidance of hereditary illnesses are made possible by these technologies.

3. *Machine learning and artificial intelligence (AI):* These two fields are becoming more and more significant in reproductive health. Large datasets can be analyzed by these technologies to find trends and forecast results, increasing the precision of diagnosis and treatment regimens. AI-powered solutions are being created to improve IVF procedures, help with embryo selection, and improve reproductive treatment in general.

4. *Non-Invasive Diagnostics:* Non-invasive diagnostic methods are growing in popularity because they provide safer and more practical ways to evaluate reproductive health. New methods of monitoring and diagnosing fertility-related disorders are being made possible by innovations like liquid biopsy, which examines the DNA of circulating tumors, and sophisticated imaging technology.

5. *Fertility Preservation:* Methods for preserving fertility, like freezing ovarian, sperm, and egg tissue, are getting easier to get and more dependable. These innovations preserve reproductive potential for later use while giving people the freedom to arrange their families as they see fit. For patients receiving medical therapies that may impact fertility, fertility preservation is especially crucial.

6. *natural and Integrative treatments:* It is becoming more widely acknowledged that combining natural and medical treatments might improve reproductive results. A complete strategy that addresses the mental, emotional, and spiritual facets of reproductive health is offered by combining evidence-based holistic therapies with traditional medical treatments.

Prospective Research Paths and Possible Innovations
There are a lot of exciting opportunities for discoveries and advancements in fertility research in the future. The future of fertility care is anticipated to be shaped by several exciting research areas:

1. *Stem Cell Research:* This quickly developing science has the potential to completely transform fertility treatments. In people with reduced ovarian reserve or premature ovarian failure, researchers are investigating the use of stem cells to rebuild ovarian tissue, enhance egg quality, and restore fertility. By boosting sperm production and rebuilding testicular tissue, stem cell therapies also show promise in treating male infertility.

2. *Mitochondrial Replacement treatment:* To stop the spread of mitochondrial disorders, mitochondrial replacement treatment (MRT) substitutes healthy donor mitochondria with damaged mitochondrial DNA. For those with mitochondrial diseases, this method may enhance the quality of the embryos and raise the likelihood of a healthy pregnancy.

3. *Reproductive Immunology:* Researching the immune system's function in fertility and pregnancy is the focus of this new field. Targeted medicines to improve reproductive outcomes can be developed by comprehending the effects of immunological variables on implantation, pregnancy maintenance, and recurrent pregnancy loss.

4. *Bioengineering and Tissue Engineering:* The potential of bioengineering and tissue engineering to produce artificial reproductive tissues and organs is being investigated. In order to offer those with severe reproductive difficulties new therapeutic choices, researchers are focusing on creating bioengineered ovaries, testicles, and uterine tissues.

5. *Epigenetic Therapies:* These treatments try to change how genes are expressed without changing the DNA sequence that underlies them. Scholars are examining how environmental elements, including nutrition, stress, and exposure to chemicals, impact epigenetic modifications that impact fertility. Fertility results and reproductive health could be enhanced by epigenetic treatments.

6. *Microbiome Research:* Due to its influence on reproductive health, the microbiome—the group of bacteria that live within the body—is receiving more attention. The effects of the gut, seminal, and vaginal microbiomes on fertility and pregnancy outcomes are being investigated.

New therapies and interventions may result from a better understanding of the microbiome's function in reproductive health.

Giving Readers the Tools to Take Control of Their Fertility Path

Giving readers the information, resources, and skills they need to take control of their fertility journey is crucial as we look to the future of fertility. The following important lessons will assist people and couples face motherhood with optimism and confidence:

1. Remain Informed: Making educated judgments requires keeping up with the most recent developments in holistic care and fertility treatments. To guarantee that you have access to the finest care possible, stay current on new research, medical recommendations, and available treatments.

2. Seek Personalized Care: To meet your particular fertility requirements and goals, personalized care is crucial. Create a customized reproductive plan that takes your situation and preferences into account by collaborating with medical professionals and holistic practitioners.

3. Take a comprehensive Approach: Take a comprehensive approach to reproductive health, including its physical, emotional, and spiritual facets. To enhance your general well-being, include dietary modifications, stress reduction strategies, lifestyle alterations, and holistic therapies.

4. Speak Up for Yourself: Speak up for your fertility and well-being. Ask questions, be open with your healthcare providers, and, if necessary, get second views. Take an active role in your reproductive journey and arm yourself with knowledge.

5. Seek Emotional Support: Getting emotional support is crucial because the fertility process can be emotionally taxing. Make connections with loved ones who can relate to your experiences, counselors, and support groups. A positive outlook and emotional fortitude are essential for managing the highs and lows of conception.

6. Examine Other Routes to Parenthood: Be willing to investigate alternate routes to parenthood, including donor gametes, adoption, and surrogacy. These choices provide you with more chances to start a family and fulfill your desire to become a parent.

7. Preserve Hope and Resilience: During the fertility process, hope and resilience are strong allies. Develop an optimistic outlook, acknowledge minor victories, and draw strength from your fortitude. Keep in mind that every person and couple's path to motherhood is different and that holding onto hope can make all the difference.

In conclusion, there are a lot of fascinating opportunities and prospective innovations in the field of fertility in the future. People and couples can take control of their reproductive journey by being knowledgeable, obtaining individualized care, adopting a holistic approach, and arming themselves with information and support. A thorough and balanced approach to fertility is provided by the fusion of contemporary science and holistic care, giving everyone hoping to start a family hope and opportunity. Future research and developments could influence the state of reproductive health for future generations as we continue to improve our knowledge and management of fertility.

With appreciation,
Dr. Elvira S. Graves

Kindly Drop a positive review for this book online, if you got value from it.
Thank you.
You can also check out my other books through this link…
https://www.amazon.com/author/elvygraves